Detox Smoothies for Your Health

Tasty Smoothie Recipes for a Total Body Detox

BY: Allie Allen

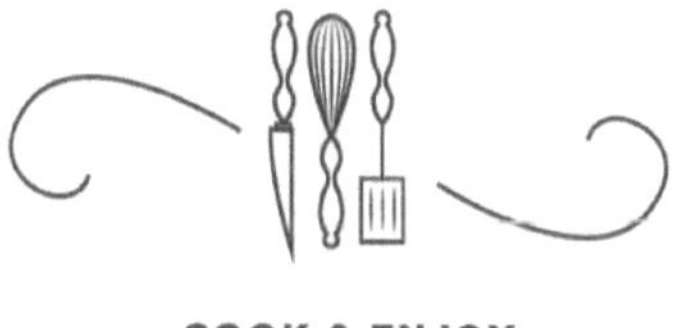

Copyright 2019 Allie Allen

Copyright Notes

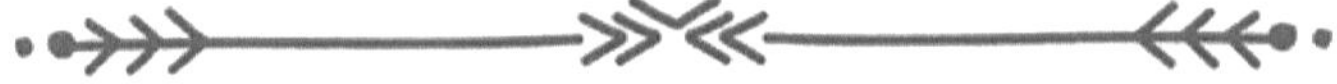

My Gift to You for Buying My Book!

I would like to extend an exclusive offer to receive free and discounted eBooks every day! This special gift is my way of saying thanks. If you fill in the subscription box below you will begin to receive special offers directly to your email.

Not only that! You will also receive notifications letting you know when an offer will expire. You will never miss a chance to get a free book! Who wouldn't want that?

Fill in the subscriber information below and get started today!

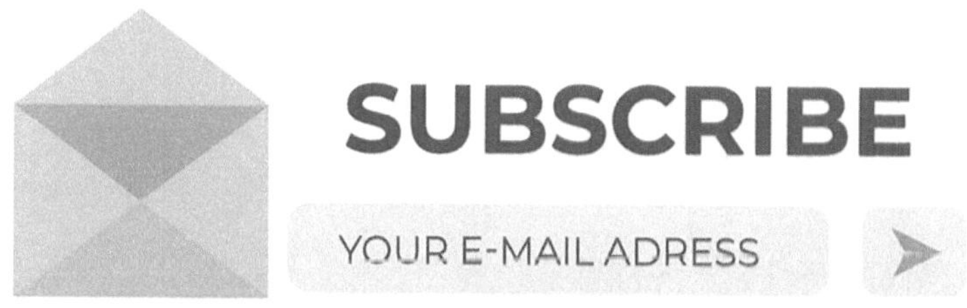

https://allie-allen.getresponsepages.com/

Table of Contents

Tasty Detox Smoothie Recipes

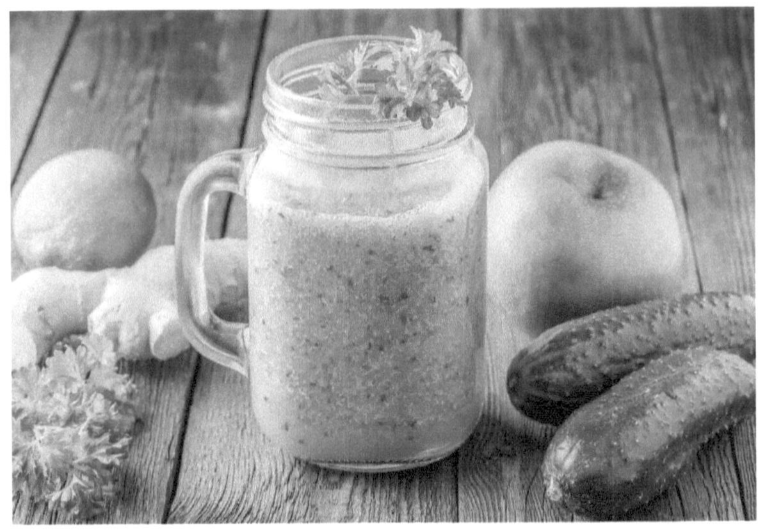

ssssssssssssssssssssssssssssssssssssssssssssssssssssss

1) Avocado Green Smoothie

Yield: 1 to 2

Creamy and delicious, this avocado green smoothie combines the nutritional power of ripe avocado and leafy greens all in one recipe.

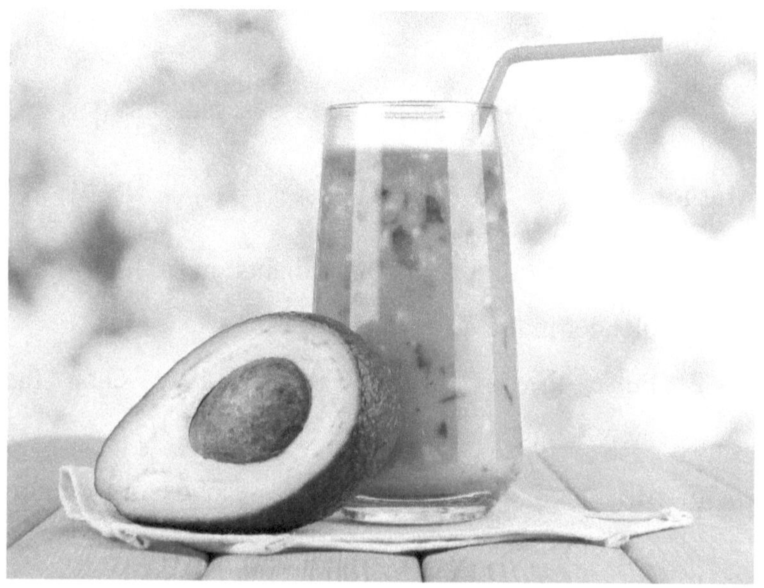

List of Ingredients:

- 1 large ripe avocado, pitted and chopped
- 1 large leaf romaine lettuce, chopped
- 1 large leaf kale, chopped
- 1 medium stalk celery, chopped
- 1 cup unsweetened almond milk
- ½ cup ice cubes
- 1 tsp. honey

sssssssssssssssssssssssssssssssssssssssssssssssssssss

Methods:

1. Combine all of the ingredients in a high-speed blender in the order listed.
2. Pulse the mixture several times to chop the ingredients.
3. Blend on high speed for 60 seconds or so until smooth.
4. Add more liquid, if desired, to thin – add ice to thicken.
5. Pour into glasses and serve immediately.

2) Kick-Start Kale Smoothie

Yield: 1 to 2

Dark, leafy kale is one of the healthiest things you can put into your body – it is so full of nutrients that it is often referred to as a "super food".

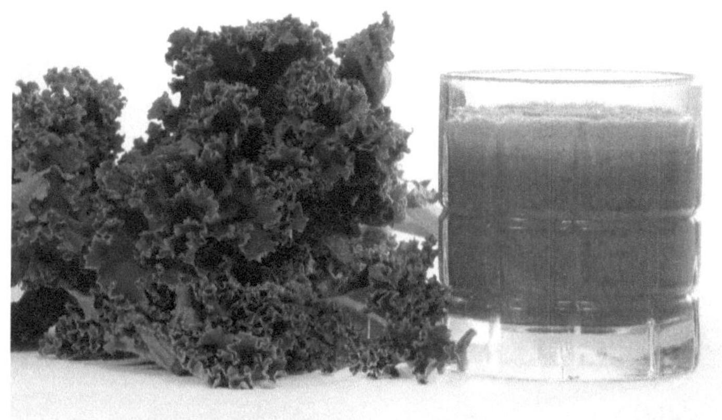

List of Ingredients:

- 2 cups fresh chopped kale
- 1 large stalk celery, chopped
- 1 medium carrot, peeled and diced
- 1 cup water or apple juice
- ½ cup ice cubes
- 1 tbsp. honey

sssssssssssssssssssssssssssssssssssssssssssssssssssss

Methods:

1. Combine all of the ingredients in a high-speed blender in the order listed.
2. Pulse the mixture several times to chop the ingredients.
3. Blend on high speed for 60 seconds or so until smooth.
4. Add more liquid, if desired, to thin – add ice to thicken.
5. Pour into glasses and serve immediately.

3) Cucumber Apple Smoothie

Yield: 1 to 2

Crunchy cucumbers and crisp apples come together in this recipe to form a delicious detox smoothie that will leave your skin glowing.

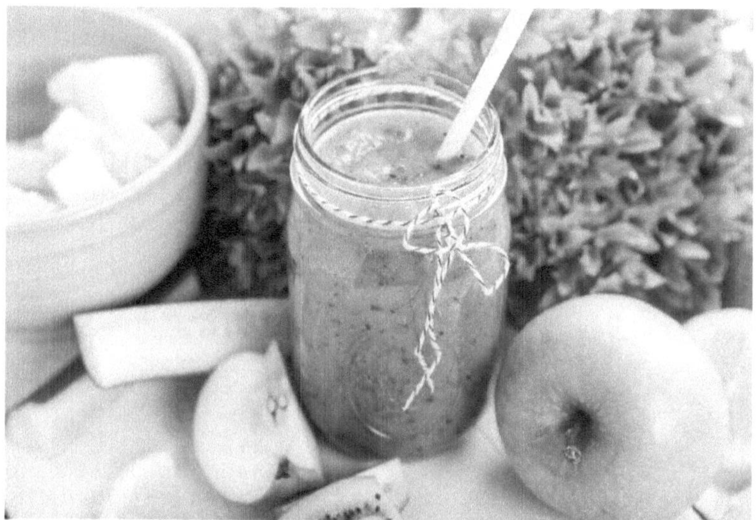

List of Ingredients:

- 1 large seedless cucumber, peeled and diced
- 2 medium ripe apples, cored and chopped
- 1 cup organic apple juice
- ½ cup ice cubes
- Pinch ground cinnamon

sssssssssssssssssssssssssssssssssssssssssssssssssssssss

Methods:

1. Combine all of the ingredients in a high-speed blender in the order listed.
2. Pulse the mixture several times to chop the ingredients.
3. Blend on high speed for 60 seconds or so until smooth.
4. Add more liquid, if desired, to thin – add ice to thicken.
5. Pour into glasses and serve immediately.

4) Sweet Red Raspberry Smoothie

Yield: 1 to 2

This sweet red raspberry smoothie is a delicious and refreshing combination of tart raspberries, smooth almond milk and honey.

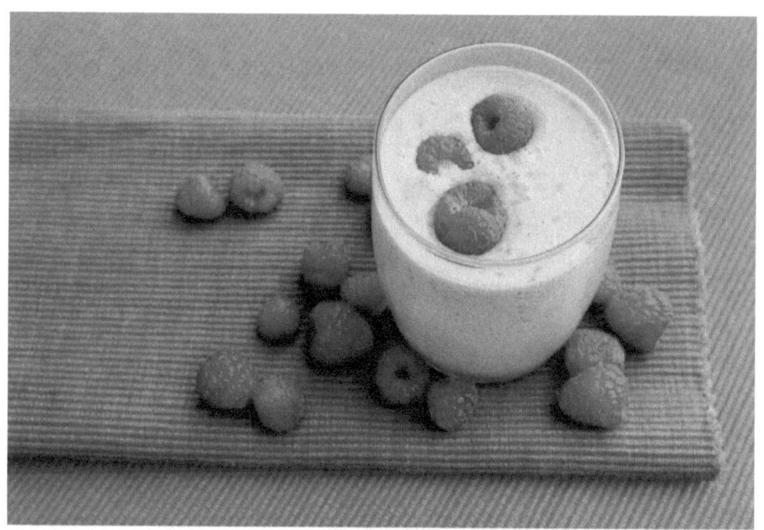

List of Ingredients:

- 2 cups frozen raspberries
- 1 large leaf kale, chopped
- 1 cup unsweetened almond milk
- 2 small stalks celery, chopped
- 1 tsp. honey

ssssssssssssssssssssssssssssssssssssssssssssssssssssss

Methods:

1. Combine all of the ingredients in a high-speed blender in the order listed.
2. Pulse the mixture several times to chop the ingredients.
3. Blend on high speed for 60 seconds or so until smooth.
4. Add more liquid, if desired, to thin – add ice to thicken.
5. Pour into glasses and serve immediately.

5) Broccoli Cucumber Smoothie

Yield: 1 to 2

All of the nutritional power of a bowl of steamed veggies brought together in a single shippable beverage – what more could you ask for?

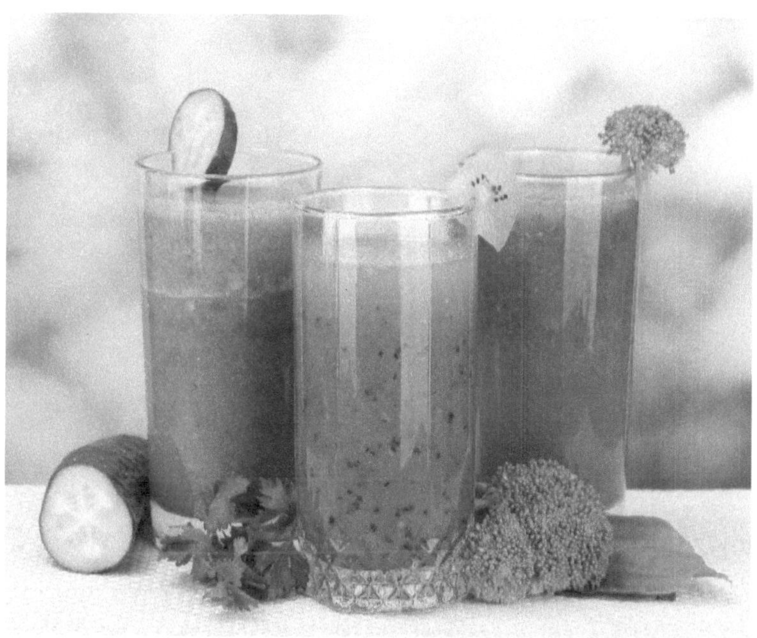

List of Ingredients:

- 1 large seedless cucumber, peeled and diced
- 1 cup chopped broccoli florets
- 1 mediums talk celery, chopped
- 1 cup organic apple juice
- ½ cup ice cubes
- 1 tsp. honey

sssssssssssssssssssssssssssssssssssssssssssssssssss

Methods:

1. Combine all of the ingredients in a high-speed blender in the order listed.
2. Pulse the mixture several times to chop the ingredients.
3. Blend on high speed for 60 seconds or so until smooth.
4. Add more liquid, if desired, to thin – add ice to thicken.
5. Pour into glasses and serve immediately.

6) Power-Packed Spinach Smoothie

Yield: 1 to 2

Spinach is packed with essential vitamins and minerals that, in combination with the other powerful ingredients in this recipe, will get you revved up and ready for your day.

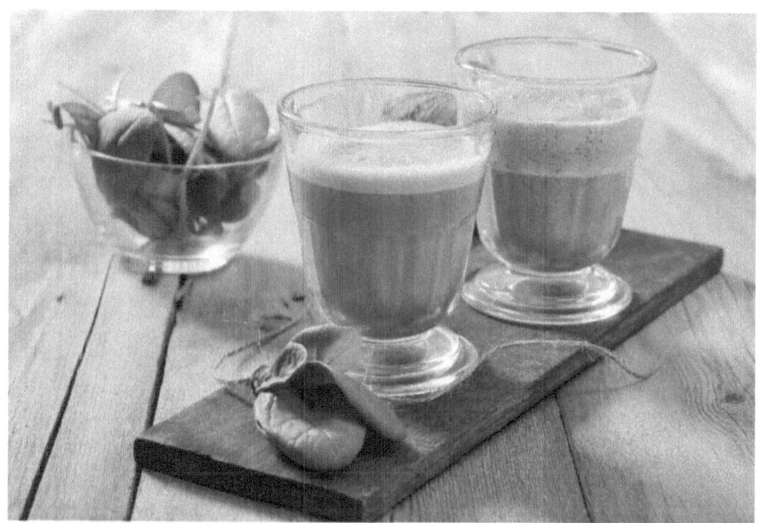

List of Ingredients:

- 2 cups fresh baby spinach, packed
- 1 large stalk celery, chopped
- ½ small seedless cucumber, chopped
- 1 cup ice cubes
- ½ cup plain Greek yogurt
- 1 tsp. dried spirulina powder

sssssssssssssssssssssssssssssssssssssssssssssssssssss

Methods:

1. Combine all of the ingredients in a high-speed blender in the order listed.
2. Pulse the mixture several times to chop the ingredients.
3. Blend on high speed for 60 seconds or so until smooth.
4. Add more liquid, if desired, to thin – add ice to thicken.
5. Pour into glasses and serve immediately.

7) Strawberry Basil Smoothie

Yield: 1 to 2

Strawberries are loaded with essential vitamins and minerals which, in combination with the nutrient power of fresh basil, makes this one healthy smoothie.

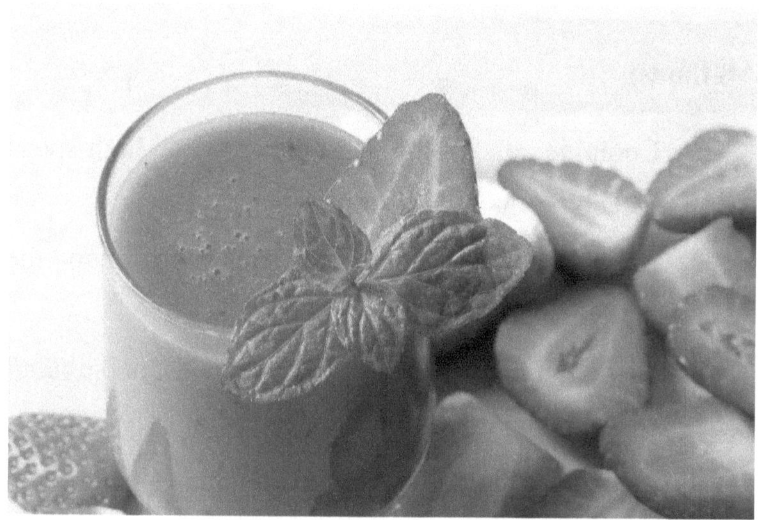

List of Ingredients:

- 2 cups frozen sliced strawberries
- ½ cup fresh chopped basil leaves
- 1 cup unsweetened almond milk
- ½ cup ice cubes
- 1 tsp. honey

sssssssssssssssssssssssssssssssssssssssssssssssssssssss

Methods:

1. Combine all of the ingredients in a high-speed blender in the order listed.
2. Pulse the mixture several times to chop the ingredients.
3. Blend on high speed for 60 seconds or so until smooth.
4. Add more liquid, if desired, to thin – add ice to thicken.
5. Pour into glasses and serve immediately.

8) Strawberry Banana Smoothie

Yield: 1 to 2

A classic combination of flavors, this strawberry banana smoothie is sure to become a family favorite in your house.

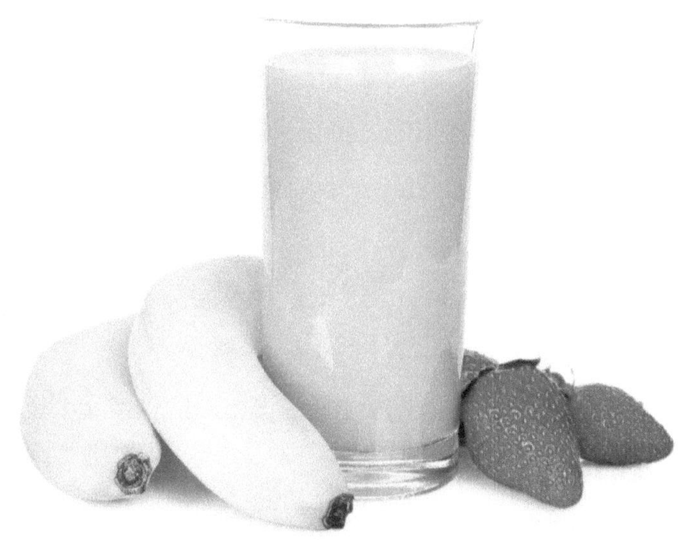

List of Ingredients:

- 2 medium frozen bananas, peeled and sliced
- 1 cup frozen sliced strawberries
- 1 cup unsweetened almond milk
- ½ cup ice cubes
- 1 tsp. honey

sssssssssssssssssssssssssssssssssssssssssssssssssss

Methods:

1. Combine all of the ingredients in a high-speed blender in the order listed.
2. Pulse the mixture several times to chop the ingredients.
3. Blend on high speed for 60 seconds or so until smooth.
4. Add more liquid, if desired, to thin – add ice to thicken.
5. Pour into glasses and serve immediately.

9) Cinnamon Banana Smoothie

Yield: 1 to 2

This cool and creamy smoothie is so delicious that you may forget it is good for you!

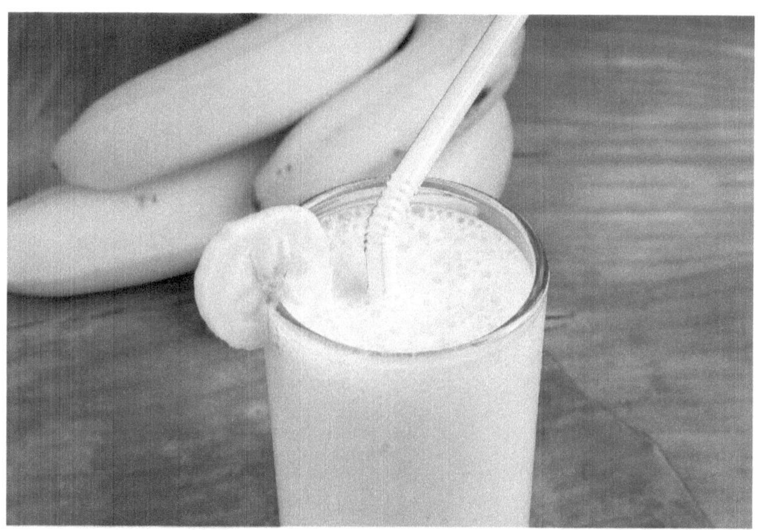

List of Ingredients:

- 2 large frozen bananas, peeled and chopped
- 1 cup unsweetened coconut milk
- ½ cup ice cubes
- ¼ tsp. ground cinnamon
- 2 drops vanilla extract

ssssssssssssssssssssssssssssssssssssssssssssssssssss

Methods:

1. Combine all of the ingredients in a high-speed blender in the order listed.
2. Pulse the mixture several times to chop the ingredients.
3. Blend on high speed for 60 seconds or so until smooth.
4. Add more liquid, if desired, to thin – add ice to thicken.
5. Pour into glasses and serve immediately.

10) Ginger Beet Smoothie

Yield: 1 to 2

When you think of your favorite vegetables, beets may not come to mind. You will be glad to know, however, that they are packed with powerful nutrients – so drink up!

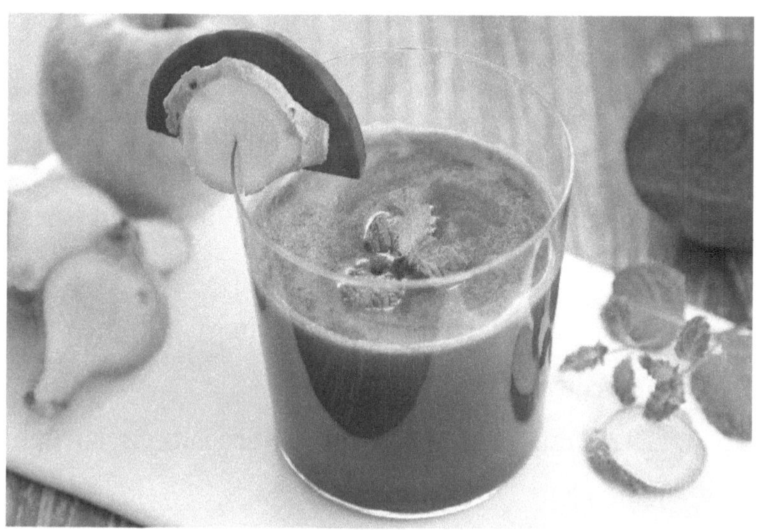

List of Ingredients:

- 1 cup fresh baby spinach
- 1 medium beet, scrubbed and chopped
- 1 tbsp. fresh minced ginger
- Juice from 1 lemon
- 1 cup ice cubes
- ½ cup organic apple juice

sssssssssssssssssssssssssssssssssssssssssssssssssss

Methods:

1. Combine all of the ingredients in a high-speed blender in the order listed.
2. Pulse the mixture several times to chop the ingredients.
3. Blend on high speed for 60 seconds or so until smooth.
4. Add more liquid, if desired, to thin – add ice to thicken.
5. Pour into glasses and serve immediately.

11) Apple Ginger Smoothie

Yield: 1 to 2

This delicious smoothie is almost like a beverage version of apple pie – it is full of fresh apple flavor and spiced with fresh ginger.

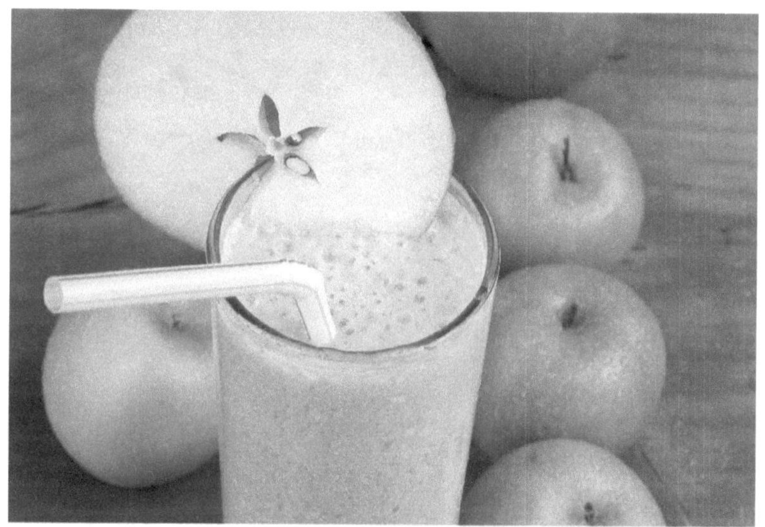

List of Ingredients:

- 2 medium ripe apples, cored and chopped
- 1 large stalk celery, chopped
- 1 medium carrot, peeled and diced
- 1 cup water or apple juice
- ½ cup ice cubes
- 1 tbsp. fresh minced ginger

ssssssssssssssssssssssssssssssssssssssssssssssssss

Methods:

1. Combine all of the ingredients in a high-speed blender in the order listed.
2. Pulse the mixture several times to chop the ingredients.
3. Blend on high speed for 60 seconds or so until smooth.
4. Add more liquid, if desired, to thin – add ice to thicken.
5. Pour into glasses and serve immediately.

12) Merry Mango Smoothie

Yield: 1 to 2

This recipe is naturally sweet, made with frozen chopped mango and flavored with organic orange juice. Enjoy this smoothie outside on a hot day.

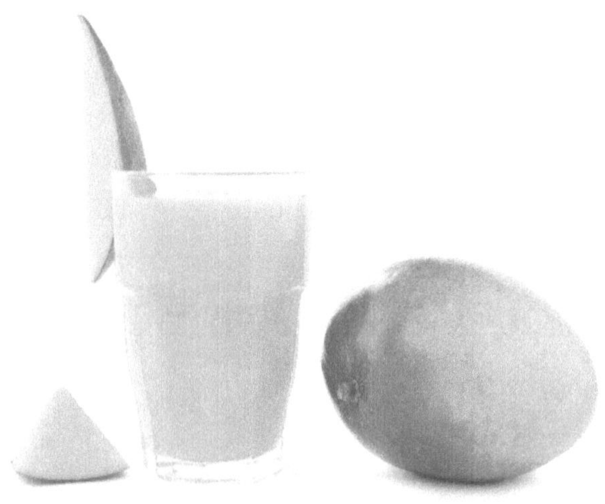

List of Ingredients:

- 2 cups frozen chopped mango
- 2 large leaves romaine lettuce, chopped
- 1 small carrot, peeled and chopped
- 1 cup organic orange juice
- ½ cup ice cubes
- 1 tbsp. fresh lemon juice

sssssssssssssssssssssssssssssssssssssssssssssssssssssss

Methods:

1. Combine all of the ingredients in a high-speed blender in the order listed.
2. Pulse the mixture several times to chop the ingredients.
3. Blend on high speed for 60 seconds or so until smooth.
4. Add more liquid, if desired, to thin – add ice to thicken.
5. Pour into glasses and serve immediately.

13) Spiced Nectarine Smoothie

Yield: 1 to 2

Nectarines are those fruits you find in the grocery store next to the peaches – they often go ignored but after tasting this recipe just once they will always have a space in your shopping cart.

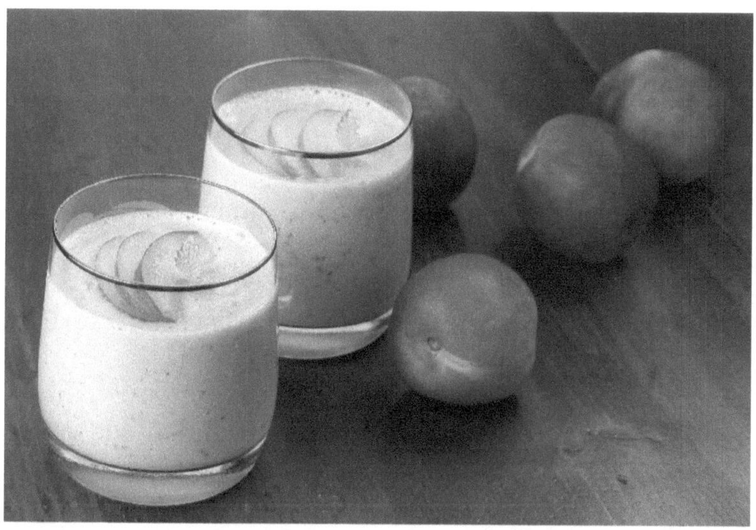

List of Ingredients:

- 2 ripe nectarines, pitted and chopped
- 1 cup unsweetened almond milk
- ½ cup ice cubes
- ¼ cup plain Greek yogurt
- Pinch ground cinnamon

sssssssssssssssssssssssssssssssssssssssssssssssss

Methods:

1. Combine all of the ingredients in a high-speed blender in the order listed.
2. Pulse the mixture several times to chop the ingredients.
3. Blend on high speed for 60 seconds or so until smooth.
4. Add more liquid, if desired, to thin – add ice to thicken.
5. Pour into glasses and serve immediately.

14) Creamy Blueberry Dream Smoothie

Yield: 1 to 2

Blueberries are incredibly high in antioxidants which help to heal your cells from free-radical damage – they may also help reduce your risk for cancer.

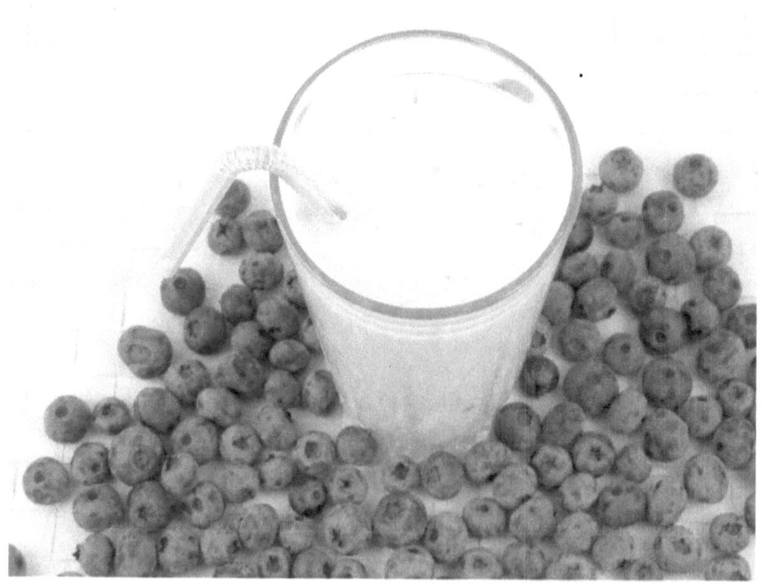

List of Ingredients:

- 2 cups frozen blueberries
- 1 large leaf kale, chopped
- 1 large stalk celery, chopped
- 1 cup unsweetened coconut milk
- ½ cup ice cubes
- 1 tsp. honey

ssssssssssssssssssssssssssssssssssssssssssssssssss

Methods:

1. Combine all of the ingredients in a high-speed blender in the order listed.
2. Pulse the mixture several times to chop the ingredients.
3. Blend on high speed for 60 seconds or so until smooth.
4. Add more liquid, if desired, to thin – add ice to thicken.
5. Pour into glasses and serve immediately.

15) Tropical Fruit Smoothie

Yield: 1 to 2

This smoothie is the perfect blend of all your favorite tropical fruits – tender banana, sweet mango and even pineapple!

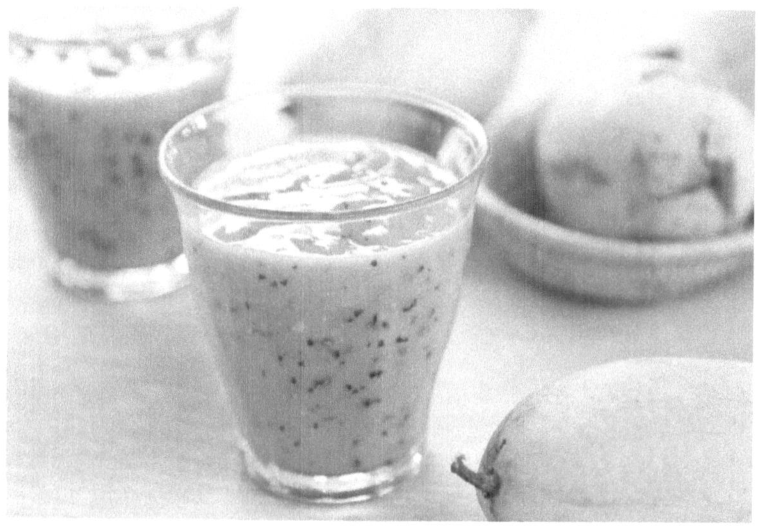

List of Ingredients:

- 1 medium frozen banana, peeled and sliced
- 1 cup frozen chopped mango
- ½ cup frozen chopped pineapple
- 1 cup organic orange juice
- ½ cup ice cubes

sssssssssssssssssssssssssssssssssssssssssssssssssss

Methods:

1. Combine all of the ingredients in a high-speed blender in the order listed.
2. Pulse the mixture several times to chop the ingredients.
3. Blend on high speed for 60 seconds or so until smooth.
4. Add more liquid, if desired, to thin – add ice to thicken.
5. Pour into glasses and serve immediately.

16) Carrot Cucumber Smoothie

Yield: 1 to 2

Two crunchy vegetables come together in this recipe to form a creamy and delicious smoothie that is positively packed with nutrients.

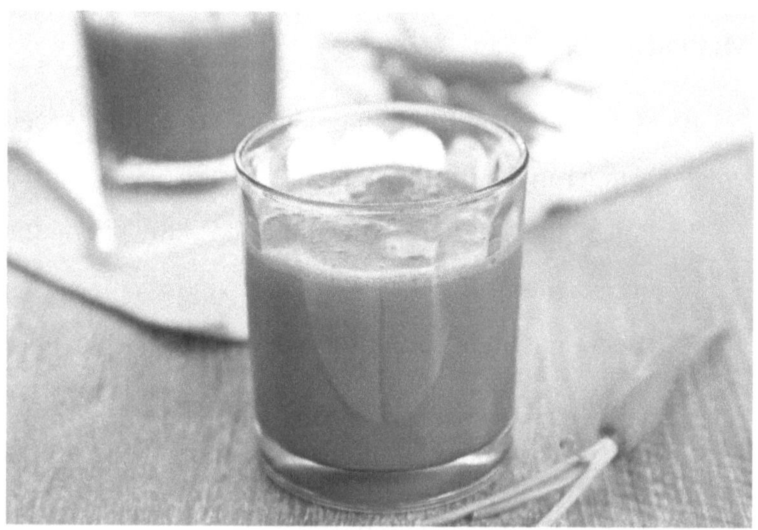

List of Ingredients:

- 1 large seedless cucumber, peeled and chopped
- 2 medium carrots, peeled and diced
- 1 large stalk celery, diced
- 1 cup organic apple juice
- ½ cup ice cubes
- Pinch ground ginger

sssssssssssssssssssssssssssssssssssssssssssssssssss

Methods:

1. Combine all of the ingredients in a high-speed blender in the order listed.
2. Pulse the mixture several times to chop the ingredients.
3. Blend on high speed for 60 seconds or so until smooth.
4. Add more liquid, if desired, to thin – add ice to thicken.
5. Pour into glasses and serve immediately.

17) Strawberry Kiwi Smoothie

Yield: 1 to 2

Two sweet and flavorful fruits come together in this creamy smoothie to provide your body with healthy nutrients and detoxification power.

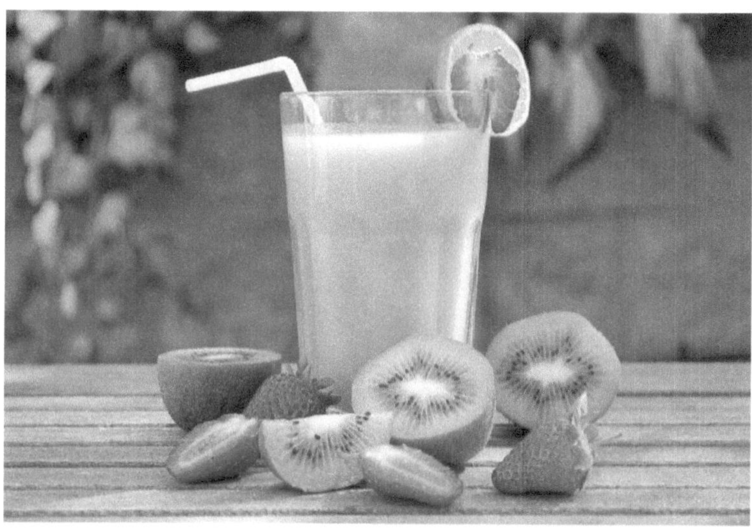

List of Ingredients:

- 2 cups frozen sliced strawberries
- 1 ripe kiwi, peeled and sliced
- 1 cup unsweetened coconut milk
- 1 tbsp. chia seeds
- 1 tsp. honey

ssssssssssssssssssssssssssssssssssssssssssssssssss

Methods:

1. Combine all of the ingredients in a high-speed blender in the order listed.
2. Pulse the mixture several times to chop the ingredients.
3. Blend on high speed for 60 seconds or so until smooth.
4. Add more liquid, if desired, to thin – add ice to thicken.
5. Pour into glasses and serve immediately.

18) Sweet Citrus Smoothie

Yield: 1 to 2

All of your favorite citrus fruits come together in this sweet and tart smoothie – feel free to sweeten it with a natural sweetener like honey, if you desire.

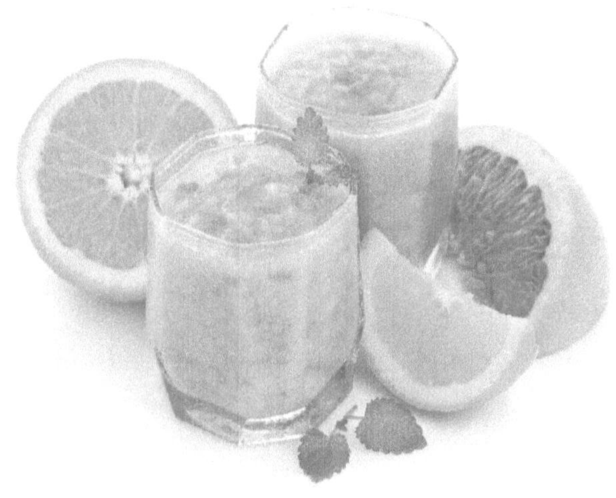

List of Ingredients:

- 2 navel oranges, peeled and chopped
- 1 cup pink grapefruit juice
- 1 cup ice cubes
- 1 tbsp. fresh lemon juice
- 1 tbsp. honey

sssssssssssssssssssssssssssssssssssssssssssssssssssss

Methods:

1. Combine all of the ingredients in a high-speed blender in the order listed.
2. Pulse the mixture several times to chop the ingredients.
3. Blend on high speed for 60 seconds or so until smooth.
4. Add more liquid, if desired, to thin – add ice to thicken.
5. Pour into glasses and serve immediately.

19) Super Celery Smoothie

Yield: 1 to 2

Celery has very high water content which is essential for a good detox – water helps to flush toxins from your system and rehydrates you so your body can function at its best.

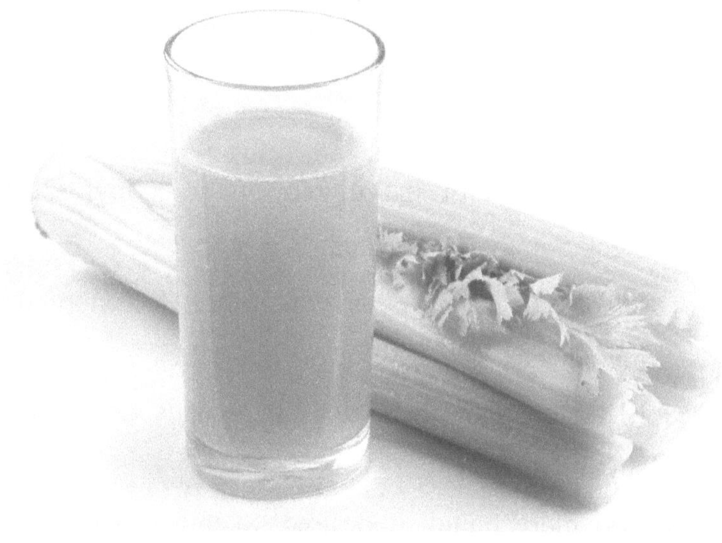

List of Ingredients:

- 3 medium stalks celery, diced
- 1 small ripe apple, cored and chopped
- ½ small seedless cucumber, peeled and diced
- ½ cup unsweetened apple juice
- 1 tbsp. ground flaxseed
- 1 tsp. fresh lemon juice

sssssssssssssssssssssssssssssssssssssssssssssssssss

Methods:

1. Combine all of the ingredients in a high-speed blender in the order listed.
2. Pulse the mixture several times to chop the ingredients.
3. Blend on high speed for 60 seconds or so until smooth.
4. Add more liquid, if desired, to thin – add ice to thicken.
5. Pour into glasses and serve immediately.

20) Avocado Walnut Smoothie

Yield: 1 to 2

Smooth avocado and crunchy walnuts make for a unique and flavorful smoothie.

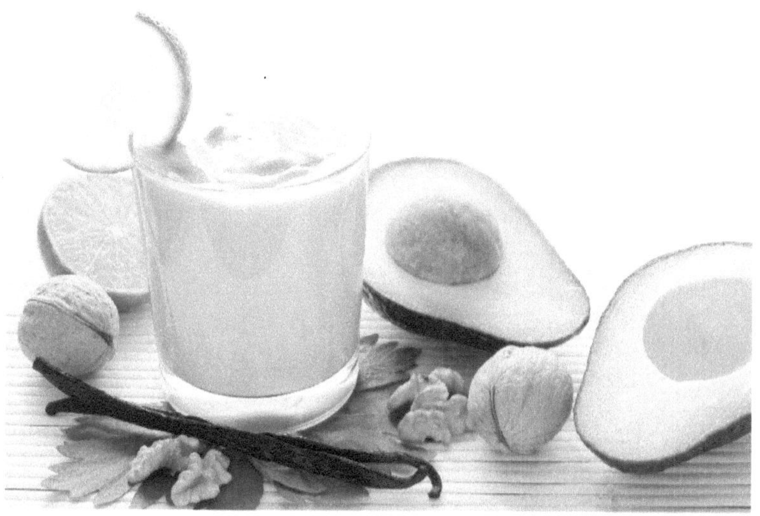

List of Ingredients:

- 1 large ripe avocado, pitted and chopped
- 2 large leaves kale, chopped
- 1 cup unsweetened almond milk
- 2 tbsp. chopped walnuts
- 1 tsp. honey

sssssssssssssssssssssssssssssssssssssssssssssssssssss

Methods:

1. Combine all of the ingredients in a high-speed blender in the order listed.
2. Pulse the mixture several times to chop the ingredients.
3. Blend on high speed for 60 seconds or so until smooth.
4. Add more liquid, if desired, to thin – add ice to thicken.
5. Pour into glasses and serve immediately.

21) Avocado Lime Smoothie

Yield: 1 to 2

The smooth and delicious flavor of ripe avocado is perfectly complemented by the tartness of fresh lime juice in this avocado lime smoothie.

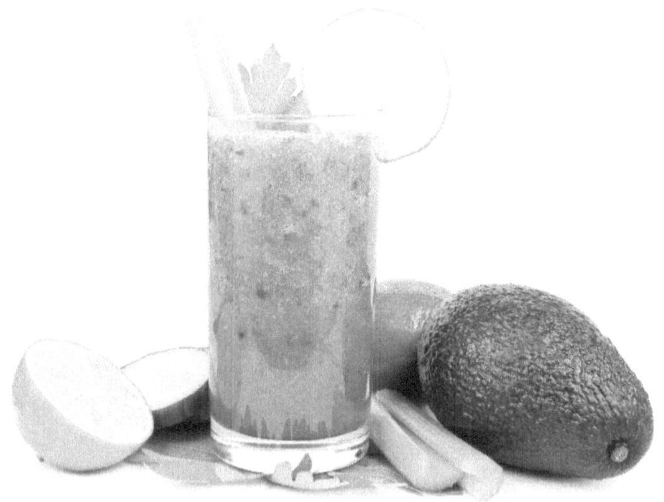

List of Ingredients:

- 1 large ripe avocado, pitted and diced
- 1 cup unsweetened almond milk
- Juice from 1 lime
- 1 tsp. lime zest
- 1 tsp. honey

sssssssssssssssssssssssssssssssssssssssssssssssssss

Methods:

1. Combine all of the ingredients in a high-speed blender in the order listed.
2. Pulse the mixture several times to chop the ingredients.
3. Blend on high speed for 60 seconds or so until smooth.
4. Add more liquid, if desired, to thin – add ice to thicken.
5. Pour into glasses and serve immediately.

22) Carrot Apple Smoothie

Yield: 1 to 2

Two of your favorite health foods combined into one recipe make for a tasty smoothie that will quickly become your go-to.

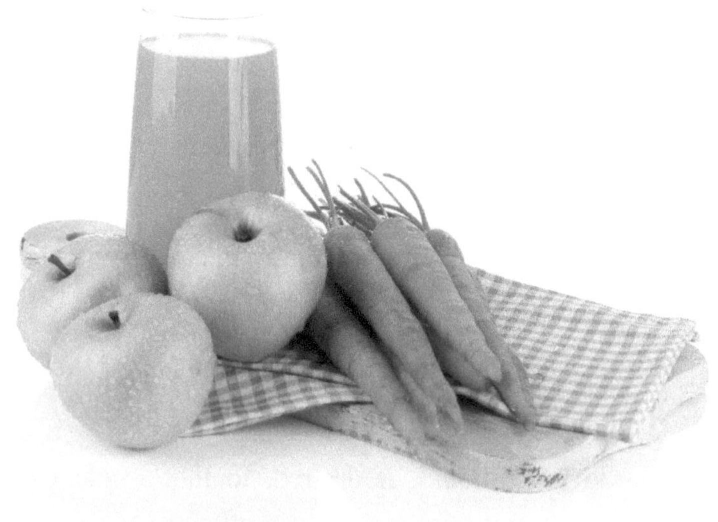

List of Ingredients:

- 3 medium carrots, peeled and diced
- 2 medium ripe apples, cored and chopped
- 1 cup unsweetened almond milk
- ½ cup ice cubes
- 1 tsp. fresh lemon juice
- Pinch ground ginger

ssssssssssssssssssssssssssssssssssssssssssssssssssss

Methods:

1. Combine all of the ingredients in a high-speed blender in the order listed.
2. Pulse the mixture several times to chop the ingredients.
3. Blend on high speed for 60 seconds or so until smooth.
4. Add more liquid, if desired, to thin – add ice to thicken.
5. Pour into glasses and serve immediately.

23) Orange Carrot Smoothie with Ginger

Yield: 1 to 2

Oranges and carrots come together in this recipe, flavored with fresh ginger – you may not know it, but ginger is full of healthy nutrients.

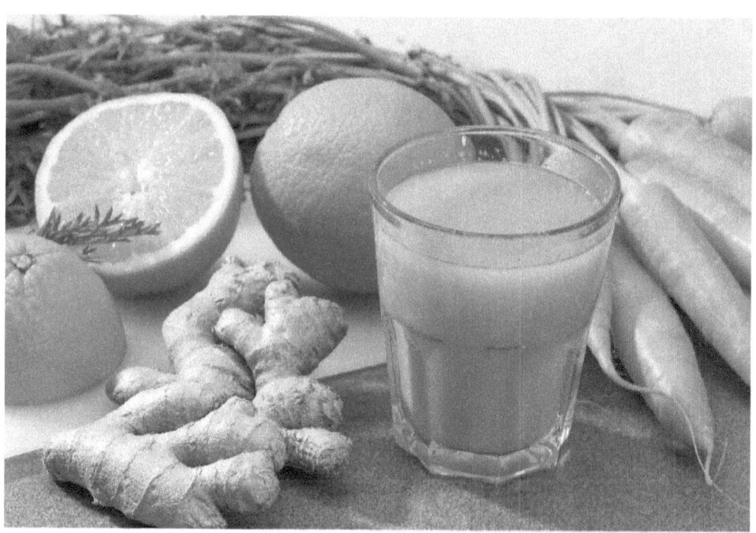

List of Ingredients:

- 2 large carrots, peeled and chopped
- 1 large navel orange, peeled and chopped
- 1 cup unsweetened almond milk
- 1 tbsp. fresh minced ginger
- 1 tsp. honey

sssssssssssssssssssssssssssssssssssssssssssssssss

Methods:

1. Combine all of the ingredients in a high-speed blender in the order listed.
2. Pulse the mixture several times to chop the ingredients.
3. Blend on high speed for 60 seconds or so until smooth.
4. Add more liquid, if desired, to thin – add ice to thicken.
5. Pour into glasses and serve immediately.

24) Green Grape Smoothie

Yield: 1 to 2

Have some extra grapes on hand? Throw them into your blender with a frozen banana and a handful of spinach to make this delicious green grape smoothie.

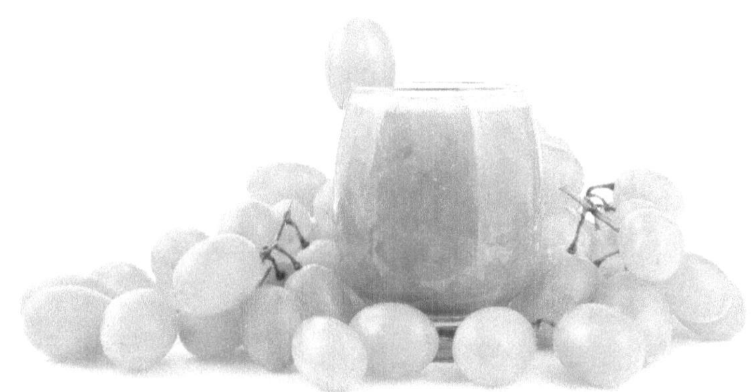

List of Ingredients:

- 1 cup green seedless grapes
- 1 frozen banana, peeled and chopped
- 1 cup fresh baby spinach
- ½ cup organic apple juice
- 1 tbsp. ground flaxseed

ssssssssssssssssssssssssssssssssssssssssssssssssssssss

Methods:

1. Combine all of the ingredients in a high-speed blender in the order listed.
2. Pulse the mixture several times to chop the ingredients.
3. Blend on high speed for 60 seconds or so until smooth.
4. Add more liquid, if desired, to thin – add ice to thicken.
5. Pour into glasses and serve immediately.

About the Author

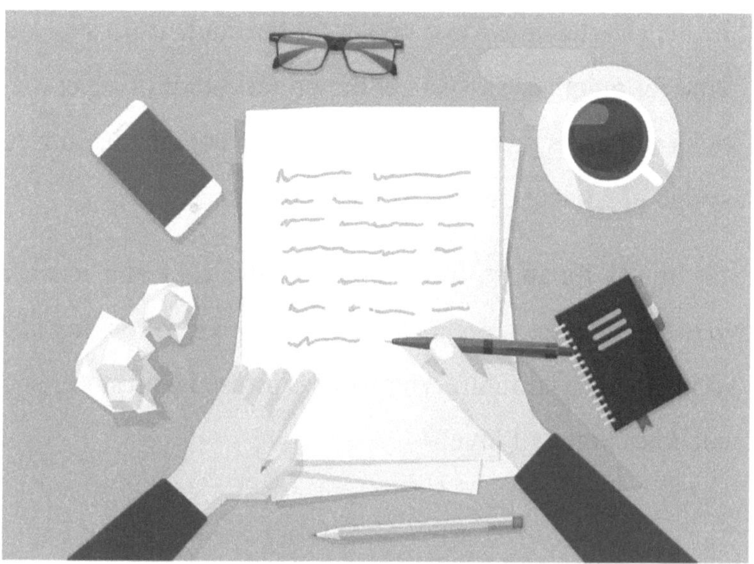

Allie Allen developed her passion for the culinary arts at the tender age of five when she would help her mother cook for their large family of 8. Even back then, her family knew this would be more than a hobby for the young Allie and when she graduated from high school, she applied to cooking school in London. It had always been a dream of the young chef to study with some of Europe's best and she made it happen by attending the Chef Academy of London.

After graduation, Allie decided to bring her skills back to North America and open up her own restaurant. After 10 successful years as head chef and owner, she decided to sell her business and pursue other career avenues. This monumental decision led Allie to her true calling, teaching. She also started to write e-books for her students to study at home for practice. She is now the proud author of several e-books and gives private and semi-private cooking lessons to a range of students at all levels of experience.

Stay tuned for more from this dynamic chef and teacher when she releases more informative e-books on cooking and baking in the near future. Her work is infused with stores and anecdotes you will love!

Author's Afterthoughts

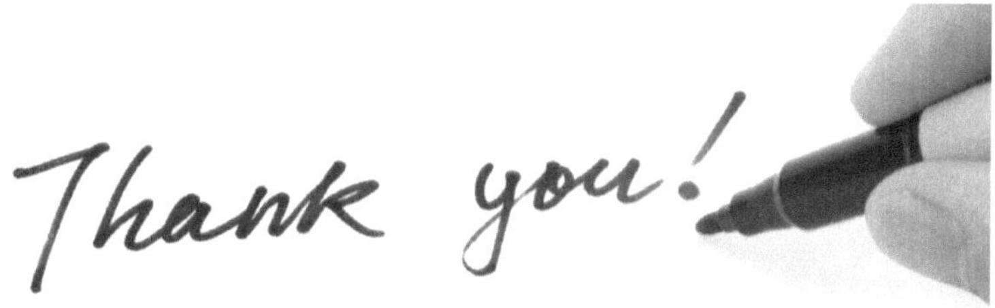

I can't tell you how grateful I am that you decided to read my book. My most heartfelt thanks that you took time out of your life to choose my work and I hope you find benefit within these pages.

There are so many books available today that offer similar content so that makes it even more humbling that you decided to buying mine.

Tell me what you thought! I am eager to hear your opinion and ideas on what you read as are others who are looking for a good book to buy. Leave a review on Amazon.com so others can benefit from your wisdom!

With much thanks,

Allie Allen